My Mediterranean Recipe Book

Don't Miss These Quick And Easy Recipes To Make Incredible Mediterranean Appetizers

Dan Peterson

TABLE OF CONTENT

Sicilian Cannellini Beans and Escarole

Preparation time: 15 minutes

Cooking time: 21 minutes

Servings: 4

INGREDIENTS:

- 1 tablespoon extra-virgin olive oil, plus extra for serving
- 2 onions, chopped fine
- Salt and pepper, to taste
- 4 garlic cloves, minced
- 1/8 teaspoon red pepper flakes
- 1 (1-pound / 454-g) head escarole, trimmed and sliced 1 inch thick
- 1 (15-ounce / 425-g) can cannellini beans, rinsed
- 1 cup chicken or vegetable broth
- 1 cup water
- 2 teaspoons lemon juice

DIRECTIONS:

Heat oil in Dutch oven over medium heat until shimmering. Add onions and ½ teaspoon salt and cook until softened and lightly browned, 5 to 7 minutes.

Stir in garlic and pepper flakes and cook until fragrant, about 30 seconds. Stir in escarole, beans, broth, and water and bring to simmer.

Cook, stirring occasionally, until escarole is wilted, about 5 minutes. Increase heat to high and cook until liquid is nearly evaporated, 10 to 15 minutes.

Stir in lemon juice and season with salt and pepper to taste. Drizzle with extra oil and serve.

NUTRITION: Calories: 110 Carbs: 18g Fat: 2g Protein: 5g

Cannellini Bean Salad

Preparation time: 15 minutes

Cooking time: 8 minutes

Servings: 6-8

INGREDIENTS:

    ¼ cup extra-virgin olive oil
    3 garlic cloves, peeled and smashed
    2 (15-ounce / 425-g) cans cannellini beans, rinsed
    Salt and pepper, to taste
    2 teaspoons sherry vinegar
    1 small shallot, minced
    1 red bell pepper, stemmed, seeded, and cut into ¼-inch pieces
    ¼ cup chopped fresh parsley
    2 teaspoons chopped fresh chives

DIRECTIONS:

Cook 1 tablespoon oil and garlic in medium saucepan over medium heat, stirring often, until garlic turns golden but not brown, about 3 minutes.

Add beans, 2 cups water, and 1 teaspoon salt and bring to simmer. Remove from heat, cover, and let sit for 20 minutes.

Meanwhile, combine vinegar and shallot in large bowl and let sit for 20 minutes. Drain beans and remove garlic.

Add beans, remaining 3 tablespoons oil, bell pepper, parsley, and chives to shallot mixture and gently toss to combine. Season with salt and pepper to taste. Let sit for 20 minutes.

Serve.

NUTRITION: Calories: 200 Carbs: 11g Fat: 14g Protein: 10g

Cannellini Bean Lettuce Wraps

Preparation time: 15 minutes

Cooking time: 10 minutes

Servings: 4

INGREDIENTS:

- 1 tablespoon extra-virgin olive oil
- ½ cup diced red onion (about ¼ onion)
- ¾ cup chopped fresh tomatoes (about 1 medium tomato)
- ¼ teaspoon freshly ground black pepper
- 1 (15-ounce) can cannellini or great northern beans, drained and rinsed
- ¼ cup finely chopped fresh curly parsley
- ½ cup Lemony Garlic Hummus or ½ cup prepared hummus
- 8 romaine lettuce leaves

DIRECTIONS:

In a large skillet over medium heat, heat the oil. Add the onion and cook for 3 minutes, stirring occasionally.

Add the tomatoes and pepper and cook for 3 more minutes, stirring occasionally. Add the beans and cook for 3 more minutes, stirring occasionally. Remove from the heat, and mix in the parsley.

Spread 1 tablespoon of hummus over each lettuce leaf. Evenly spread the warm bean mixture down the center of each leaf.

Fold one side of the lettuce leaf over the filling lengthwise, then fold over the other side to make a wrap and serve.

NUTRITION: Calories: 211 Fat: 8g Carbohydrates: 28g Protein: 10g

Israeli Eggplant, Chickpea, and Mint Sauté

Preparation time: 5 minutes

Cooking time: 20 minutes

Servings: 6

INGREDIENTS:
- Nonstick cooking spray
- 1 medium globe eggplant (about 1 pound), stem removed
- 1 tablespoon extra-virgin olive oil
- 2 tablespoons freshly squeezed lemon juice (from about 1 small lemon)
- 2 tablespoons balsamic vinegar
- 1 teaspoon ground cumin
- ¼ teaspoon kosher or sea salt
- 1 (15-ounce) can chickpeas, drained and rinsed
- 1 cup sliced sweet onion (about ½ medium Walla Walla or Vidalia onion)
- ¼ cup loosely packed chopped or torn mint leaves
- 1 tablespoon sesame seeds, toasted if desired
- 1 garlic clove, finely minced (about ½ teaspoon)

DIRECTIONS:
- Place one oven rack about 4 inches below the broiler element. Turn the broiler to the highest setting to preheat. Spray a large, rimmed baking sheet with nonstick cooking spray.
- On a cutting board, cut the eggplant lengthwise into four slabs (each piece should be about ½- to 1/8-inch thick). Place the eggplant slabs on

the prepared baking sheet. Set aside.

In a small bowl, whisk together the oil, lemon juice, vinegar, cumin, and salt. Brush or drizzle 2 tablespoons of the lemon dressing over both sides of the eggplant slabs. Reserve the remaining dressing.

Broil the eggplant directly under the heating element for 4 minutes, flip them, then broil for another 4 minutes, until golden brown.

While the eggplant is broiling, in a serving bowl, combine the chickpeas, onion, mint, sesame seeds, and garlic. Add the reserved dressing, and gently mix to incorporate all the ingredients.

When the eggplant is done, using tongs, transfer the slabs from the baking sheet to a cooling rack and cool for 3 minutes.

When slightly cooled, place the eggplant on a cutting board and slice each slab crosswise into ½-inch strips.

Add the eggplant to the serving bowl with the onion mixture. Gently toss everything together, and serve warm or at room temperature.

NUTRITION: Calories: 159 Fat: 4g Carbohydrates: 26g Protein: 6g

Mediterranean Lentils and Rice

Preparation time : 5 minutes
Cooking time : 25 minutes

Servings: 4

INGREDIENTS:

- 2¼ cups low-sodium or no-salt-added vegetable broth
- ½ cup uncooked brown or green lentils
- ½ cup uncooked instant brown rice
- ½ cup diced carrots (about 1 carrot)
- ½ cup diced celery (about 1 stalk)
- 1 (2.25-ounce) can sliced olives, drained (about ½ cup)
- ¼ cup diced red onion (about 1/8 onion)
- ¼ cup chopped fresh curly-leaf parsley
- 1½ tablespoons extra-virgin olive oil
- 1 tablespoon freshly squeezed lemon juice (from about ½ small lemon)
- 1 garlic clove, minced (about ½ teaspoon)
- ¼ teaspoon kosher or sea salt
- ¼ teaspoon freshly ground black pepper

DIRECTIONS:

In a medium saucepan over high heat, bring the broth and lentils to a boil, cover, and lower the heat to medium-low. Cook for 8 minutes.

Raise the heat to medium, and stir in the rice. Cover the pot and cook the mixture for 15 minutes, or until the liquid is absorbed. Remove the pot from the heat and let it sit, covered, for 1 minute, then stir.

While the lentils and rice are cooking, mix together the carrots, celery, olives, onion, and parsley in a large serving bowl.

In a small bowl, whisk together the oil, lemon juice, garlic, salt, and pepper. Set aside. When the lentils and rice are cooked, add them to the serving bowl.

Pour the dressing on top, and mix everything together. Serve warm or cold, or store in a sealed container in the refrigerator for up to 7 days.

NUTRITION: Calories: 230 Fat: 8g Carbohydrates: 34g Protein: 8g

Brown Rice Pilaf with Golden Raisins

Preparation time: 5 minutes

Cooking time: 15 minutes

Servings: 6

INGREDIENTS:

    1 tablespoon extra-virgin olive oil
    1 cup chopped onion (about ½ medium onion)
    ½ cup shredded carrot (about 1 medium carrot)
    1 teaspoon ground cumin
    ½ teaspoon ground cinnamon
    2 cups instant brown rice
    1¾ cups 100% orange juice
    ¼ cup water
    1 cup golden raisins
    ½ cup shelled pistachios
    Chopped fresh chives (optional)

DIRECTIONS:

In a medium saucepan over medium-high heat, heat the oil. Add the onion and cook for 5 minutes, stirring frequently.

Add the carrot, cumin, and cinnamon, and cook for 1 minute, stirring frequently. Stir in the rice, orange juice, and water.

Bring to a boil, cover, then lower the heat to medium-low. Simmer for 7 minutes, or until the rice is cooked through and the liquid is absorbed. Stir in the raisins, pistachios, and chives (if using) and serve.

NUTRITION: Calories: 320 Fat: 7g Carbohydrates: 61g
Protein: 6g

Quinoa and Chickpea Vegetable Bowls

Preparation time: 15 minutes

Cooking time: 15 minutes

Servings : 4

INGREDIENTS:

- 1 cup red dry quinoa, rinsed and drained
- 2 cups low-sodium vegetable soup
- 2 cups fresh spinach
- 2 cups finely shredded red cabbage
- 1 (15-ounce / 425-g) can chickpeas, drained and rinsed
- 1 ripe avocado, thinly sliced
- 1 cup shredded carrots
- 1 red bell pepper, thinly sliced
- 4 tablespoons Mango Sauce
- ½ cup fresh cilantro, chopped
- Mango Sauce:
- 1 mango, diced
- ¼ cup fresh lime juice
- ½ teaspoon ground turmeric
- 1 teaspoon finely minced fresh ginger
- ¼ teaspoon sea salt
- Pinch of ground red pepper
- 1 teaspoon pure maple syrup
- 2 tablespoons extra-virgin olive oil

DIRECTIONS:

Pour the quinoa and vegetable soup in a saucepan. Bring to a boil. Reduce the heat to low. Cover and cook for 15 minutes or until tender. Fluffy with a fork.

Meanwhile, combine the ingredients for the mango sauce in a food processor. Pulse until smooth.

Divide the quinoa, spinach, and cabbage into 4 serving bowls, then top with chickpeas, avocado, carrots, and bell pepper.

Dress them with the mango sauce and spread with cilantro. Serve immediately.

NUTRITION: Calories: 366 Fat: 11.1g Protein: 15.5g Carbs: 55.6g

Ritzy Veggie Chili

Preparation time: 15 minutes

Cooking time : 5 hours

Servings: 4

INGREDIENTS:
- 1 (28-ounce / 794-g) can chopped tomatoes, with the juice
- 1 (15-ounce / 425-g) can black beans, drained and rinsed
- 1 (15-ounce / 425-g) can redly beans, drained and rinsed
- 1 medium green bell pepper, chopped
- 1 yellow onion, chopped
- 1 tablespoon onion powder
- 1 teaspoon paprika
- 1 teaspoon cayenne pepper
- 1 teaspoon garlic powder
- ½ teaspoon sea salt
- ½ teaspoon ground black pepper
- 1 tablespoon olive oil
- 1 large hass avocado, pitted, peeled, and chopped, for garnish

DIRECTIONS:
Combine all the ingredients, except for the avocado, in the slow cooker. Stir to mix well.

Put the slow cooker lid on and cook on high for 5 hours or until the vegetables are tender and the mixture has a thick consistency.

Pour the chili in a large serving bowl. Allow to cool for 30 minutes, then spread with chopped

avocado and serve.
NUTRITION: Calories: 633 Fat: 16.3g Protein: 31.7g
Carbs: 97.0g

Spicy Italian Bean Balls with Marinara

Preparation time: 15 minutes

Cooking time: 30 minutes

Servings: 2-4

INGREDIENTS:

Bean Balls:
1 tablespoon extra-virgin olive oil
½ yellow onion, minced
1 teaspoon fennel seeds
2 teaspoons dried oregano
½ teaspoon crushed red pepper flakes
1 teaspoon garlic powder
1 (15-ounce / 425-g) can white beans (cannellini or navy), drained and rinsed
½ cup whole-grain bread crumbs
Sea salt and ground black pepper, to taste
Marinara:
1 tablespoon extra-virgin olive oil
3 garlic cloves, minced
Handful basil leaves
1 (28-ounce / 794-g) can chopped tomatoes with juice reserved
Sea salt, to taste

DIRECTIONS:

Preheat the oven to 350°F (180°C). Line a baking sheet with parchment paper. Heat the olive oil in a nonstick skillet over medium heat until shimmering.

Add the onion and sauté for 5 minutes or until translucent. Sprinkle with fennel seeds, oregano, red pepper flakes, and garlic powder, then cook for 1 minute or until aromatic.

Pour the sautéed mixture in a food processor and add the beans and bread crumbs. Sprinkle with salt and ground black pepper, then pulse to combine well and the mixture holds together.

Shape the mixture into balls with a 2-ounce (57-g) cookie scoop, then arrange the balls on the baking sheet.

Bake in the preheated oven for 30 minutes or until lightly browned. Flip the balls halfway through the cooking time.

While baking the bean balls, heat the olive oil in a saucepan over medium-high heat until shimmering. Add the garlic and basil and sauté for 2 minutes or until fragrant.

Fold in the tomatoes and juice. Bring to a boil. Reduce the heat to low. Put the lid on and simmer for 15 minutes. Sprinkle with salt.

Transfer the bean balls on a large plate and baste with marinara before serving.

NUTRITION: Calories: 351 Fat: 16.4g Protein: 11.5g Carbs: 42.9g

Baked Rolled Oat with Pears and Pecans

Preparation time: 15 minutes

Cooking time: 30 minutes

Servings: 6

INGREDIENTS:

- 2 tablespoons coconut oil, melted, plus more for greasing the pan
- 3 ripe pears, cored and diced
- 2 cups unsweetened almond milk
- 1 tablespoon pure vanilla extract
- ¼ cup pure maple syrup
- 2 cups gluten-free rolled oats
- ½ cup raisins
- ¾ cup chopped pecans
- ¼ teaspoon ground nutmeg
- 1 teaspoon ground cinnamon
- ½ teaspoon ground ginger
- ¼ teaspoon sea salt

DIRECTIONS:

Preheat the oven to 350ºF (180ºC). Grease a baking dish with melted coconut oil, then spread the pears in a single layer on the baking dish evenly.

Combine the almond milk, vanilla extract, maple syrup, and coconut oil in a bowl. Stir to mix well.

Combine the remaining ingredients in a separate large bowl. Stir to mix well. Fold the almond milk mixture in the bowl, then pour the mixture over the pears.

Place the baking dish in the preheated oven and bake for 30 minutes or until lightly browned and set. Serve immediately.

NUTRITION: Calories: 479 Fat: 34.9g Protein: 8.8g Carbs: 50.1g

Brown Rice Pilaf with Pistachios and Raisins

Preparation time: 15 minutes

Cooking time: 15 minutes

Servings: 6

INGREDIENTS:

- 1 tablespoon extra-virgin olive oil
- 1 cup chopped onion
- ½ cup shredded carrot
- ½ teaspoon ground cinnamon
- 1 teaspoon ground cumin
- 2 cups brown rice
- 1¾ cups pure orange juice
- ¼ cup water
- ½ cup shelled pistachios
- 1 cup golden raisins
- ½ cup chopped fresh chives

DIRECTIONS:

Heat the olive oil in a saucepan over medium-high heat until shimmering. Add the onion and sauté for 5 minutes or until translucent.

Add the carrots, cinnamon, and cumin, then sauté for 1 minutes or until aromatic.

Pour int the brown rice, orange juice, and water. Bring to a boil. Reduce the heat to medium-low and simmer for 7 minutes or until the liquid is almost absorbed.

Transfer the rice mixture in a large serving bowl, then spread with pistachios, raisins, and chives. Serve immediately.

NUTRITION: Calories: 264 Fat: 7.1g Protein: 5.2g Carbs: 48.9g

Cherry, Apricot, and Pecan Brown Rice Bowl

Preparation time: 15 minutes
Cooking time: 1 hour & 1 minute

Servings: 2

INGREDIENTS:

      2 tablespoons olive oil
      2 green onions, sliced
      ½ cup brown rice
      1 cup low -sodium chicken stock
      2 tablespoons dried cherries
      4 dried apricots, chopped
      2 tablespoons pecans, toasted and chopped
      Sea salt and freshly ground pepper, to taste

DIRECTIONS:

Heat the olive oil in a medium saucepan over medium-high heat until shimmering. Add the green onions and sauté for 1 minutes or until fragrant.

Add the rice. Stir to mix well, then pour in the chicken stock. Bring to a boil. Reduce the heat to low. Cover and simmer for 50 minutes or until the brown rice is soft.

Add the cherries, apricots, and pecans, and simmer for 10 more minutes or until the fruits are tender.

Pour them in a large serving bowl. Fluff with a fork. Sprinkle with sea salt and freshly ground pepper. Serve immediately.

NUTRITION: Calories: 451 Fat: 25.9g Protein: 8.2g
Carbs: 50.4g

Curry Apple Couscous with Leeks and Pecans

Preparation time: 15 minutes

Cooking time: 8 minutes

Servings: 4

INGREDIENTS:

2 teaspoons extra-virgin olive oil
2 leeks, white parts only, sliced
1 apple, diced
2 cups cooked couscous
2 tablespoons curry powder
½ cup chopped pecans

DIRECTIONS:

Heat the olive oil in a skillet over medium heat until shimmering. Add the leeks and sauté for 5 minutes or until soft.

Add the diced apple and cook for 3 more minutes until tender. Add the couscous and curry powder. Stir to combine. Transfer them in a large serving bowl, then mix in the pecans and serve.

NUTRITION: Calories: 254 Fat: 11.9g Protein: 5.4g Carbs: 34.3g

Lebanese Flavor Broken Thin Noodles

Preparation time: 15 minutes

Cooking time: 25 minutes

Servings: 6

INGREDIENTS:

- 1 tablespoon extra-virgin olive oil
- 1 (3-ounce / 85-g) cup vermicelli, broken into 1- to 1½-inch pieces
- 3 cups shredded cabbage
- 1 cup brown rice
- 3 cups low-sodium vegetable soup
- ½ cup water
- 2 garlic cloves, mashed
- ¼ teaspoon sea salt
- 1/8 teaspoon crushed red pepper flakes
- ½ cup coarsely chopped cilantro
- Fresh lemon slices, for serving

DIRECTIONS:

Heat the olive oil in a saucepan over medium-high heat until shimmering. Add the vermicelli and sauté for 3 minutes or until toasted. Add the cabbage and sauté for 4 minutes or until tender.

Pour in the brown rice, vegetable soup, and water. Add the garlic and sprinkle with salt and red pepper flakes.

Bring to a boil over high heat. Reduce the heat to medium low. Put the lid on and simmer for

another 10 minutes. Turn off the heat, then let
sit for 5 minutes without opening the lid.

Pour them on a large serving platter and spread
with cilantro. Squeeze the lemon slices over
and serve warm.

NUTRITION: Calories: 127 Fat: 3.1g Protein: 4.2g Carbs:
22.9g

Lemony Farro and Avocado Bowl

Preparation time: 1 5 minutes

Cooking time: 25 minutes

Servings : 4

INGREDIENTS:
- 1 tablespoon plus 2 teaspoons extra-virgin olive oil, divided
- ½ medium onion, chopped
- 1 carrot, shredded
- 2 garlic cloves, minced
- 1 (6-ounce / 170-g) cup pearled farro
- 2 cups low-sodium vegetable soup
- 2 avocados, peeled, pitted, and sliced
- Zest and juice of 1 small lemon
- ¼ teaspoon sea salt

DIRECTIONS:
- Heat 1 tablespoon of olive oil in a saucepan over medium-high heat until shimmering. Add the onion and sauté for 5 minutes or until translucent. Add the carrot and garlic and sauté for 1 minute or until fragrant.
- Add the farro and pour in the vegetable soup. Bring to a boil over high heat. Reduce the heat to low. Put the lid on and simmer for 20 minutes or until the farro is al dente.
- Transfer the farro in a large serving bowl, then fold in the avocado slices. Sprinkle with lemon zest and salt, then drizzle with lemon juice and

2 teaspoons of olive oil. Stir to mix well and
serve immediately.

NUTRITION: Calories: 210 Fat: 11.1g Protein: 4.2g
Carbs: 27.9g

Rice and Blueberry Stuffed Sweet Potatoes

Preparation time: 15 minutes

Cooking time: 20 minutes

Servings : 4

INGREDIENTS:
- 2 cups cooked wild rice
- ½ cup dried blueberries
- ½ cup chopped hazelnuts
- ½ cup shredded Swiss chard
- 1 teaspoon chopped fresh thyme
- 1 scallion, white and green parts, peeled and thinly sliced
- Sea salt and freshly ground black pepper, to taste
- 4 sweet potatoes, baked in the skin until tender

DIRECTIONS:
- Preheat the oven to 400ºF (205ºC). Combine all the ingredients, except for the sweet potatoes, in a large bowl. Stir to mix well.
- Cut the top third of the sweet potato off length wire, then scoop most of the sweet potato flesh out. Fill the potato with the wild rice mixture, then set the sweet potato on a greased baking sheet.
- Bake in the preheated oven for 20 minutes or until the sweet potato skin is lightly charred. Serve immediately.

NUTRITION: Calories: 393 Fat: 7.1g Protein: 10.2g Carbs: 76.9g

Farro Salad Mix

Preparation time: 15 minutes

Cooking time: 33 minutes

Servings: 4-6

INGREDIENTS:

1 teaspoon Dijon mustard

1½ cups whole farro

2 ounces feta cheese, crumbled (½ cup)

2 tablespoons lemon juice

2 tablespoons minced shallot

3 tablespoons chopped fresh dill

3 tablespoons extra-virgin olive oil

6 ounces asparagus, trimmed and cut into 1-inch lengths

6 ounces cherry tomatoes, halved

6 ounces sugar snap peas, strings removed, cut into 1-inch lengths

Salt and pepper

DIRECTIONS:

Bring 4 quarts water to boil in a Dutch oven. Put in asparagus, snap peas, and 1 tablespoon salt and cook until crisp-tender, approximately 3 minutes.

Use a slotted spoon to move vegetables to large plate and allow to cool completely, about 15 minutes. Put in farro to water, return to boil, and cook until grains are soft with slight chew, 15 to 30 minutes.

Drain farro, spread in rimmed baking sheet, and allow to cool completely, about 15 minutes.

Beat oil, lemon juice, shallot, mustard, ¼ teaspoon salt, and ¼ teaspoon pepper together in a big container.

Put in vegetables, farro, tomatoes, dill, and ¼ cup feta and toss gently to combine. Sprinkle with salt and pepper to taste. Move to serving platter and drizzle with remaining ¼ cup feta. Serve.

NUTRITION: Calories: 240 Carbs: 26g Fat: 12g Protein: 9g

Farrotto Mix

Preparation time: 15 minutes

Cooking time: 40 minutes

Servings: 6

INGREDIENTS:

½ onion, chopped fine

1 cup frozen peas, thawed

1 garlic clove, minced

1 tablespoon minced fresh chives

1 teaspoon grated lemon zest plus 1 teaspoon juice

1½ cups whole farro

1½ ounces Parmesan cheese, grated (¾ cup)

2 tablespoons extra-virgin olive oil

2 teaspoons minced fresh tarragon

3 cups chicken broth

3 cups water

4 ounces asparagus, trimmed and cut on bias into 1-inch lengths

4 ounces pancetta, cut into ¼-inch pieces

Salt and pepper

DIRECTIONS:

Pulse farro using a blender until about half of grains are broken into smaller pieces, about 6 pulses.

Bring broth and water to boil in moderate-sized saucepan on high heat. Put in asparagus and cook until crisp-tender, 2 to 3 minutes.

Use a slotted spoon to move asparagus to a container and set aside. Decrease heat to low, cover broth mixture, and keep warm.

Cook pancetta in a Dutch oven on moderate heat until lightly browned and fat has rendered, approximately 5 minutes.

Put in 1 tablespoon oil and onion and cook till they become tender, approximately 5 minutes. Mix in garlic and cook until aromatic, approximately half a minute.

Put in farro and cook, stirring often, until grains are lightly toasted, approximately three minutes.

Stir 5 cups warm broth mixture into farro mixture, decrease the heat to low, cover, and cook until almost all liquid has been absorbed and farro is just al dente, about 25 minutes, stirring twice during cooking.

Put in peas, tarragon, ¾ teaspoon salt, and ½ teaspoon pepper and cook, stirring continuously, until farro becomes creamy, approximately 5 minutes.

Remove from the heat, mix in Parmesan, chives, lemon zest and juice, remaining 1 tablespoon oil, and reserved asparagus.

Adjust consistency with remaining warm broth mixture as required (you may have broth left over). Sprinkle with salt and pepper to taste. Serve.

NUTRITION : Calories: 218 Carbs: 41g Fat: 2g Protein: 7g

Fennel-Parmesan Farro

Preparation time: 15 minutes

Cooking time: 50 minutes

Servings: 4-6

INGREDIENTS:

¼ cup minced fresh parsley

1 onion, chopped fine

1 ounce Parmesan cheese, grated (½ cup)

1 small fennel bulb, stalks discarded, bulb halved, cored, and chopped fine

1 teaspoon minced fresh thyme or ¼ teaspoon dried

1½ cups whole farro

2 teaspoons sherry vinegar

3 garlic cloves, minced

3 tablespoons extra-virgin olive oil

Salt and pepper

DIRECTIONS:

Bring 4 quarts water to boil in a Dutch oven. Put in farro and 1 tablespoon salt, return to boil, and cook until grains are soft with slight chew, 15 to 30 minutes.

Drain farro, return to now-empty pot, and cover to keep warm. Heat 2 tablespoons oil in 12-inch frying pan on moderate heat until it starts to shimmer.

Put in onion, fennel, and ¼ teaspoon salt and cook, stirring intermittently, till they become tender, 8 to 10 minutes. Put in garlic and thyme and cook until aromatic, approximately half a minute.

Put in residual 1 tablespoon oil and farro and cook, stirring often, until heated through, approximately 2 minutes.

Remove from the heat, mix in Parmesan, parsley, and vinegar. Sprinkle with salt and pepper to taste. Serve.

NUTRITION: Calories: 338 Carbs: 56g Fat: 10g Protein: 11g

Feta-Grape-Bulgur Salad with Grapes and Feta

Preparation time: 15 minutes

Cooking time: 1 hour & 30 minutes

Servings: 4-6

INGREDIENTS:

¼ cup chopped fresh mint

¼ cup extra-virgin olive oil

¼ teaspoon ground cumin

½ cup slivered almonds, toasted

1 cup water

1½ cups medium-grind bulgur, rinsed

2 ounces feta cheese, crumbled (½ cup)

2 scallions, sliced thin

5 tablespoons lemon juice (2 lemons)

6 ounces seedless red grapes, quartered (1 cup)

Pinch cayenne pepper

Salt and pepper

DIRECTIONS:

Mix bulgur, water, ¼ cup lemon juice, and ¼ teaspoon salt in a container. Cover and allow to sit at room temperature until grains are softened and liquid is fully absorbed, about 1½ hours.

Beat remaining 1 tablespoon lemon juice, oil, cumin, cayenne, and ¼ teaspoon salt together in a big container.

Put in bulgur, grapes, 1/3 cup almonds, 1/3 cup feta, scallions, and mint and gently toss to combine. Sprinkle with salt and pepper to taste. Sprinkle with remaining almonds and remaining feta before you serve.

NUTRITION: Calories: 500 Carbs: 45g Fat: 14g Protein: 50g

Greek Style Meaty Bulgur

Preparation time: 15 minutes

Cooking time: 30 minutes

Servings: 4-6

INGREDIENTS:

½ cup jarred roasted red peppers, rinsed, patted dry, and chopped

1 bay leaf

1 cup medium-grind bulgur, rinsed

1 onion, chopped fine

1 tablespoon chopped fresh dill

1 teaspoon extra-virgin olive oil

1 1/3 cups vegetable broth

2 teaspoons minced fresh marjoram or ½ teaspoon dried

3 garlic cloves, minced

8 ounces ground lamb

Lemon wedges

Salt and pepper

DIRECTIONS:

Heat oil in a big saucepan on moderate to high heat until just smoking. Put in lamb, ½ teaspoon salt, and ¼ teaspoon pepper and cook, breaking up meat with wooden spoon, until browned, 3 to 5 minutes.

Mix in onion and red peppers and cook until onion is softened, 5 to 7 minutes. Mix in garlic and marjoram and cook until aromatic, approximately half a minute.

Mix in bulgur, broth, and bay leaf and bring to simmer. Decrease heat to low, cover, and simmer gently until bulgur is tender, 16 to 18 minutes.

Remove from the heat, lay clean dish towel underneath lid and let bulgur sit for about 10 minutes.

Put in dill and fluff gently with fork to combine. Sprinkle with salt and pepper to taste. Serve with lemon wedges.

NUTRITION: Calories: 137 Carbs: 16g Fat: 5g Protein: 7g

Hearty Barley Mix

Preparation time: 15 minutes

Cooking time: 50 minutes

Servings: 4

INGREDIENTS:

1/8 teaspoon ground cardamom

½ cup plain yogurt

½ teaspoon ground cumin

2/3 cup raw sunflower seeds

¾ teaspoon ground coriander

1 cup pearl barley

1½ tablespoons minced fresh mint

1½ teaspoons grated lemon zest plus 1½ tablespoons juice

3 tablespoons extra-virgin olive oil

5 carrots, peeled

8 ounces snow peas, strings removed, halved along the length

Salt and pepper

DIRECTIONS:

Beat yogurt, ½ teaspoon lemon zest and 1½ teaspoons juice, 1½ teaspoons mint, ¼ teaspoon salt, and 1/8 teaspoon pepper together in a small-sized container; cover put inside your fridge until ready to serve.

Bring 4 quarts water to boil in a Dutch oven. Put in barley and 1 tablespoon salt, return to boil, and cook until tender, 20 to 40 minutes. Drain barley, return to now-empty pot, and cover to keep warm.

In the meantime, halve carrots crosswise, then halve or quarter along the length to create uniformly sized pieces.

Heat 1 tablespoon oil in 12-inch frying pan on moderate to high heat until just smoking. Put in carrots and ½ teaspoon coriander and cook, stirring intermittently, until mildly charred and just tender, 5 to 7 minutes.

Put in snow peas and cook, stirring intermittently, until spotty brown, 3 to 5 minutes; move to plate.

Heat 1½ teaspoons oil in now-empty frying pan on moderate heat until it starts to shimmer. Put in sunflower seeds, cumin, cardamom, remaining ¼ teaspoon coriander, and ¼ teaspoon salt.

Cook, stirring continuously, until seeds are toasted, approximately 2 minutes; move to small-sized container.

Beat remaining 1 teaspoon lemon zest and 1 tablespoon juice, remaining 1 tablespoon mint, and remaining 1½ tablespoons oil together in a big container.

Put in barley and carrot–snow pea mixture and gently toss to combine. Sprinkle with salt and pepper to taste. Serve, topping individual portions with spiced sunflower seeds and drizzling with yogurt sauce.

NUTRITION: Calories: 193 Carbs: 44g Fat: 1g Protein: 4g

Hearty Barley Risotto

Preparation time: 15 minutes

Cooking time: 60 minutes

Servings: 4-6

INGREDIENTS:

1 carrot, peeled and chopped fine

1 cup dry white wine

1 onion, chopped fine

1 teaspoon minced fresh thyme or ¼ teaspoon dried

1½ cups pearl barley

2 ounces Parmesan cheese, grated (1 cup)

2 tablespoons extra-virgin olive oil

4 cups chicken or vegetable broth

4 cups water

Salt and pepper

DIRECTIONS:

Bring broth and water to simmer in moderate-sized saucepan. Decrease heat to low and cover to keep warm.

Heat 1 tablespoon oil in a Dutch oven on moderate heat until it starts to shimmer. Put in onion and carrot and cook till they become tender, 5 to 7 minutes.

Put in barley and cook, stirring frequently, until lightly toasted and aromatic, about 4 minutes. Put in wine and cook, stirring often, until fully absorbed, approximately two minutes.

Mix in 3 cups warm broth and thyme, bring to simmer, and cook, stirring intermittently, until liquid is absorbed and bottom of pot is dry, 22 to 25 minutes.

Mix in 2 cups warm broth, bring to simmer, and cook, stirring intermittently, until liquid is absorbed and bottom of pot is dry, fifteen to twenty minutes.

Carry on cooking risotto, stirring frequently and adding warm broth as required to stop pot bottom from becoming dry, until barley is cooked through, 15 to 20 minutes.

Remove from the heat, adjust consistency with remaining warm broth as required. Mix in Parmesan and residual 1 tablespoon oil and sprinkle with salt and pepper to taste. Serve.

NUTRITION: Calories: 222 Carbs: 33g Fat: 5g Protein: 6g

Hearty Freekeh Pilaf

Preparation time: 15 minutes

Cooking time: 60 minutes

Servings: 4-6

INGREDIENTS:

¼ cup chopped fresh mint

¼ cup extra-virgin olive oil, plus extra for serving

¼ cup shelled pistachios, toasted and coarsely chopped

¼ teaspoon ground coriander

¼ teaspoon ground cumin

1 head cauliflower (2 pounds), cored and cut into ½-inch florets

1 shallot, minced

1½ cups whole freekeh

1½ tablespoons lemon juice

1½ teaspoons grated fresh ginger

3 ounces pitted dates, chopped (½ cup)

Salt and pepper

DIRECTIONS:

Bring 4 quarts water to boil in a Dutch oven. Put in freekeh and 1 tablespoon salt, return to boil, and cook until grains are tender, 30 to 45 minutes. Drain freekeh, return to now-empty pot, and cover to keep warm.

Heat 2 tablespoons oil in 12-inch non-stick frying pan on moderate to high heat until it starts to shimmer.

Put in cauliflower, ½ teaspoon salt, and ¼ teaspoon pepper, cover, and cook until florets are softened and start to brown, approximately five minutes.

Remove lid and continue to cook, stirring intermittently, until florets turn spotty brown, about 10 minutes.

Put in remaining 2 tablespoons oil, dates, shallot, ginger, coriander, and cumin and cook, stirring often, until dates and shallot are softened and aromatic, approximately 3 minutes.

Decrease heat to low, put in freekeh, and cook, stirring often, until heated through, about 1 minute. Remove from the heat, mix in pistachios, mint, and lemon juice.

Sprinkle with salt and pepper to taste and drizzle with extra oil. Serve.

NUTRITION: Calories: 520 Carbs: 54g Fat: 14g Protein: 36g

Herby-Lemony Farro

Preparation time: 15 minutes

Cooking time: 40 minutes

Servings : 4-6

INGREDIENTS:

¼ cup chopped fresh mint

¼ cup chopped fresh parsley

1 garlic clove, minced

1 onion, chopped fine

1 tablespoon lemon juice

1½ cups whole farro

3 tablespoons extra-virgin olive oil

Salt and pepper

DIRECTIONS:

Bring 4 quarts water to boil in a Dutch oven. Put in farro and 1 tablespoon salt, return to boil, and cook until grains are soft with slight chew, 15 to 30 minutes. Drain farro, return to now-empty pot, and cover to keep warm.

Heat 2 tablespoons oil in 12-inch frying pan on moderate heat until it starts to shimmer. Put in onion and ¼ teaspoon salt and cook till they become tender, approximately five minutes.

Mix in garlic and cook until aromatic, approximately half a minute. Put in residual 1 tablespoon oil and farro and cook, stirring often, until heated through, approximately two minutes.

Remove from the heat, mix in parsley, mint, and lemon juice. Sprinkle with salt and pepper to taste. Serve.

NUTRITION: Calories: 243 Carbs: 22g Fat: 14g Protein: 10g

Mushroom-Bulgur Pilaf

Preparation time: 15 minutes

Cooking time: 30 minutes

Servings: 4

INGREDIENTS:

¼ cup minced fresh parsley

¼ ounce dried porcini mushrooms, rinsed and minced

¾ cup chicken or vegetable broth

¾ cup water

1 cup medium-grind bulgur, rinsed

1 onion, chopped fine

2 garlic cloves, minced

2 tablespoons extra-virgin olive oil

8 ounces cremini mushrooms, trimmed, halved if small or quartered if large

Salt and pepper

DIRECTIONS:

Heat oil in a big saucepan on moderate heat until it starts to shimmer. Put in onion, porcini mushrooms, and ½ teaspoon salt and cook until onion is softened, approximately 5 minutes.

Mix in cremini mushrooms, increase heat to medium-high, cover, and cook until cremini release their liquid and begin to brown, about 4 minutes.

Mix in garlic and cook until aromatic, approximately half a minute. Mix in bulgur, broth, and water and bring to simmer.

Decrease heat to low, cover, and simmer gently until bulgur is tender, 16 to 18 minutes.

Remove from the heat, lay clean dish towel underneath lid and let pilaf sit for about ten minutes.

Put in parsley to pilaf and fluff gently with fork to combine. Sprinkle with salt and pepper to taste. Serve.

NUTRITION: Calories: 259 Carbs: 50g Fat: 3g Protein: 11g

Baked Brown Rice

Preparation time: 15 minutes
Cooking time: 1 hour & 25 minutes

Servings: 4-6

INGREDIENTS:

½ cup minced fresh parsley
¾ cup jarred roasted red peppers, rinsed, patted dry, and chopped
1 cup chicken or vegetable broth
1½ cups long-grain brown rice, rinsed
2 onions, chopped fine
2¼ cups water
4 teaspoons extra-virgin olive oil
Grated Parmesan cheese
Lemon wedges
Salt and pepper

DIRECTIONS:

Place the oven rack in the center of the oven and pre-heat your oven to 375 degrees. Heat oil in a Dutch oven on moderate heat until it starts to shimmer.

Put in onions and 1 teaspoon salt and cook, stirring intermittently, till they become tender and well browned, 12 to 14 minutes.

Mix in water and broth and bring to boil. Mix in rice, cover, and move pot to oven. Bake until rice becomes soft and liquid is absorbed, 65 to 70 minutes.

Remove pot from oven. Sprinkle red peppers over rice, cover, and allow to sit for about five minutes.

Put in parsley to rice and fluff gently with fork to combine. Sprinkle with salt and pepper to taste. Serve with grated Parmesan and lemon wedges.

NUTRITION: Calories: 100 Carbs: 27g Fat: 21g Protein: 2g

Barley Pilaf

Preparation time : 15 minutes

Cooking time: 45 minutes

Servings: 4-6

INGREDIENTS:
> ¼ cup minced fresh parsley
> 1 small onion, chopped fine
> 1½ cups pearl barley, rinsed
> 1½ teaspoons lemon juice
> 1½ teaspoons minced fresh thyme or ½ teaspoon dried
> 2 garlic cloves, minced
> 2 tablespoons minced fresh chives
> 2½ cups water
> 3 tablespoons extra-virgin olive oil
> Salt and pepper

DIRECTIONS:
> Heat oil in a big saucepan on moderate heat until it starts to shimmer. Put in onion and ½ teaspoon salt and cook till they become tender, approximately 5 minutes.
>
> Mix in barley, garlic, and thyme and cook, stirring often, until barley is lightly toasted and aromatic, approximately three minutes.
>
> Mix in water and bring to simmer. Decrease heat to low, cover, and simmer until barley becomes soft and water is absorbed, 20 to 40 minutes.
>
> Remove from the heat, lay clean dish towel underneath lid and let pilaf sit for about ten minutes. Put in parsley, chives, and lemon

juice to pilaf and fluff gently with fork to combine. Sprinkle with salt and pepper to taste. Serve.

NUTRITION: Calories: 39 Carbs: 8g Fat: 1g Protein: 1g

Basmati Rice Pilaf Mix

Preparation time: 15 minutes

Cooking time: 25 minutes

Servings: 4-6

INGREDIENTS:
- ¼ cup currants
- ¼ cup sliced almonds, toasted
- ¼ teaspoon ground cinnamon
- ½ teaspoon ground turmeric
- 1 small onion, chopped fine
- 1 tablespoon extra-virgin olive oil
- 1½ cups basmati rice, rinsed
- 2 garlic cloves, minced
- 2¼ cups water
- Salt and pepper

DIRECTIONS:
- Heat oil in a big saucepan on moderate heat until it starts to shimmer. Put in onion and ¼ teaspoon salt and cook till they become tender, approximately 5 minutes.
- Put in rice, garlic, turmeric, and cinnamon and cook, stirring often, until grain edges begin to turn translucent, approximately three minutes.
- Mix in water and bring to simmer. Decrease heat to low, cover, and simmer gently until rice becomes soft and water is absorbed, 16 to 18 minutes.
- Remove from the heat, drizzle currants over pilaf. Cover, laying clean dish towel underneath lid, and let pilaf sit for about ten minutes.

Put in almonds to pilaf and fluff gently with fork to combine. Sprinkle with salt and pepper to taste. Serve.

NUTRITION: Calories: 180 Carbs: 36g Fat: 2g Protein: 4g

Brown Rice Salad with Asparagus, Goat Cheese, and Lemon

Preparation time: 15 minutes

Cooking time: 35 minutes

Servings: 4-6

INGREDIENTS :
- ¼ cup minced fresh parsley
- ¼ cup slivered almonds, toasted
- 1 pound asparagus, trimmed and cut into 1-inch lengths
- 1 shallot, minced
- 1 teaspoon grated lemon zest plus 3 tablespoons juice
- 1½ cups long-grain brown rice
- 2 ounces goat cheese, crumbled (½ cup)
- 3½ tablespoons extra-virgin olive oil
- Salt and pepper

DIRECTIONS:

Bring 4 quarts water to boil in a Dutch oven. Put in rice and 1½ teaspoons salt and cook, stirring intermittently, until rice is tender, about half an hour.

Drain rice, spread onto rimmed baking sheet, and drizzle with 1 tablespoon lemon juice. Allow it to cool completely, about 15 minutes.

Heat 1 tablespoon oil in 12-inch frying pan on high heat until just smoking. Put in asparagus, ¼ teaspoon salt, and ¼ teaspoon pepper and cook, stirring intermittently, until asparagus is browned and crisp-tender, about 4 minutes; move to plate and allow to cool slightly.

Beat remaining 2½ tablespoons oil, lemon zest and remaining 2 tablespoons juice, shallot, ½ teaspoon salt, and ½ teaspoon pepper together in a big container.

Put in rice, asparagus, 2 tablespoons goat cheese, 3 tablespoons almonds, and 3 tablespoons parsley. Gently toss to combine and allow to sit for about 10 minutes.

Sprinkle with salt and pepper to taste. Move to serving platter and drizzle with remaining 2 tablespoons goat cheese, remaining 1 tablespoon almonds, and remaining 1 tablespoon parsley. Serve.

NUTRITION: Calories: 197 Carbs: 6g Fat: 16g Protein: 7g

Carrot-Almond-Bulgur Salad

Preparation time: 1 hour & 45 minutes

Cooking time: 0 minutes

Servings: 4-6

INGREDIENTS:
- 1/8 teaspoon cayenne pepper
- 1/3 cup chopped fresh cilantro
- 1/3 cup chopped fresh mint
- 1/3 cup extra-virgin olive oil
- ½ cup sliced almonds, toasted
- ½ teaspoon ground cumin
- 1 cup water
- 1½ cups medium-grind bulgur, rinsed
- 3 scallions, sliced thin
- 4 carrots, peeled and shredded
- 6 tablespoons lemon juice (2 lemons)
- Salt and pepper

DIRECTIONS:
- Mix bulgur, water, ¼ cup lemon juice, and ¼ teaspoon salt in a container. Cover and allow to sit at room temperature until grains are softened and liquid is fully absorbed, about 1½ hours.
- Beat remaining 2 tablespoons lemon juice, oil, cumin, cayenne, and ½ teaspoon salt together in a big container.
- Put in bulgur, carrots, scallions, almonds, mint, and cilantro and gently toss to combine. Sprinkle with salt and pepper to taste. Serve.

NUTRITION: Calories: 240 Carbs: 54g Fat: 2g Protein: 7g

Chickpea-Spinach-Bulgur

Preparation time: 15 minutes

Cooking time: 23 minutes

Servings: 4-6

INGREDIENTS:

¾ cup chicken or vegetable broth
¾ cup water
1 (15-ounce) can chickpeas, rinsed
1 cup medium-grind bulgur, rinsed
1 onion, chopped fine
1 tablespoon lemon juice
2 tablespoons za'atar
3 garlic cloves, minced
3 ounces (3 cups) baby spinach, chopped
3 tablespoons extra-virgin olive oil
Salt and pepper

DIRECTIONS:

Heat 2 tablespoons oil in a big saucepan on moderate heat until it starts to shimmer. Put in onion and ½ teaspoon salt and cook till they become tender, approximately 5 minutes.

Mix in garlic and 1 tablespoon za'atar and cook until aromatic, approximately half a minute. Mix in bulgur, chickpeas, broth, and water and bring to simmer. Decrease heat to low, cover, and simmer gently until bulgur is tender, 16 to 18 minutes.

Remove from the heat, lay clean dish towel underneath lid and let bulgur sit for about ten minutes.

Put in spinach, lemon juice, remaining 1 tablespoon za'atar, and residual 1 tablespoon oil and fluff gently with fork to combine. Sprinkle with salt and pepper to taste. Serve.

NUTRITION: Calories: 319 Carbs: 43g Fat: 12g Protein: 10g

Italian Seafood Risotto

Preparation time: 15 minutes

Cooking time: 60 minutes

Servings: 4-6

INGREDIENTS:

> 1/8 teaspoon saffron threads, crumbled
> 1 (14.5-ounce) can diced tomatoes, drained
> 1 cup dry white wine
> 1 onion, chopped fine
> 1 tablespoon lemon juice
> 1 teaspoon minced fresh thyme or ¼ teaspoon dried
> 12 ounces large shrimp (26 to 30 per pound), peeled and deveined, shells reserved
> 12 ounces small bay scallops
> 2 bay leaves
> 2 cups Arborio rice
> 2 cups chicken broth
> 2 tablespoons minced fresh parsley
> 2½ cups water
> 4 (8-ounce) bottles clam juice
> 5 garlic cloves, minced
> 5 tablespoons extra-virgin olive oil
> Salt and pepper

DIRECTIONS:

> Bring shrimp shells, broth, water, clam juice, tomatoes, and bay leaves to boil in a big saucepan on moderate to high heat. Decrease the heat to a simmer and cook for 20 minutes.

Strain mixture through fine-mesh strainer into big container, pressing on solids to extract as much liquid as possible; discard solids. Return broth to now-empty saucepan, cover, and keep warm on low heat.

Heat 2 tablespoons oil in a Dutch oven on moderate heat until it starts to shimmer. Put in onion and cook till they become tender, approximately 5 minutes.

Put in rice, garlic, thyme, and saffron and cook, stirring often, until grain edges begin to turn translucent, approximately 3 minutes.

Put in wine and cook, stirring often, until fully absorbed, approximately three minutes. Mix in 3½ cups warm broth, bring to simmer, and cook, stirring intermittently, until almost fully absorbed, about 15 minutes.

Carry on cooking rice, stirring often and adding warm broth, 1 cup at a time, every few minutes as liquid is absorbed, until rice is creamy and cooked through but still somewhat firm in center, about 15 minutes.

Mix in shrimp and scallops and cook, stirring often, until opaque throughout, approximately three minutes. Remove pot from heat, cover, and allow to sit for about 5 minutes.

Adjust consistency with remaining warm broth as required. Mix in remaining 3 tablespoons oil, parsley, and lemon juice and sprinkle with salt and pepper to taste. Serve.

NUTRITION: Calories: 450 Carbs: 12g Fat: 40g Protein: 31g

Classic Stovetop White Rice

Preparation time: 15 minutes

Cooking time: 22 minutes

Servings: 4-6

INGREDIENTS:
- 1 tablespoon extra-virgin olive oil
- 2 cups long-grain white rice, rinsed
- 3 cups water
- Basmati, jasmine, or Texmati rice can be substituted for the long-grain rice.
- Salt and pepper

DIRECTIONS:
- Heat oil in a big saucepan on moderate heat until it starts to shimmer. Put in rice and cook, stirring frequently, until grain edges begin to turn translucent, approximately 2 minutes.
- Put in water and 1 teaspoon salt and bring to simmer. Cover, decrease the heat to low, and simmer gently until rice becomes soft and water is absorbed, approximately 20 minutes.
- Remove from the heat, lay clean dish towel underneath lid and let rice sit for about ten minutes. Gently fluff rice with fork. Sprinkle with salt and pepper to taste. Serve.

NUTRITION: Calories: 160 Carbs: 36g Fat: 0g Protein: 3g

Classic Tabbouleh

Preparation time: 2 hours

Cooking time: 0 minutes

Servings: 4-6

INGREDIENTS:
- 1/8 teaspoon cayenne pepper
- ¼ cup lemon juice (2 lemons)
- ½ cup medium-grind bulgur, rinsed
- ½ cup minced fresh mint
- 1½ cups minced fresh parsley
- 2 scallions, sliced thin
- 3 tomatoes, cored and cut into ½-inch pieces
- 6 tablespoons extra-virgin olive oil
- Salt and pepper

DIRECTIONS:
Toss tomatoes with ¼ teaspoon salt using a fine-mesh strainer set over bowl and let drain, tossing occasionally, for 30 minutes; reserve 2 tablespoons drained tomato juice.

Toss bulgur with 2 tablespoons lemon juice and reserved tomato juice in a container and allow to sit until grains start to become tender, 30 to 40 minutes.

Beat remaining 2 tablespoons lemon juice, oil, cayenne, and ¼ teaspoon salt together in a big container. Put in tomatoes, bulgur, parsley, mint, and scallions and toss gently to combine.

Cover and allow to sit at room temperature until flavors have blended and bulgur is tender, about 1 hour. Before serving, toss salad to recombine and sprinkle with salt and pepper to taste.

NUTRITION: Calories: 150 Carbs: 8g Fat: 12g Protein: 4g

Farro Cucumber-Mint Salad

Preparation time: 15 minutes

Cooking time: 30 minutes

Servings: 4-6

INGREDIENTS:
- 1 cup baby arugula
- 1 English cucumber, halved along the length, seeded, and cut into ¼-inch pieces
- 1½ cups whole farro
- 2 tablespoons lemon juice
- 2 tablespoons minced shallot
- 2 tablespoons plain Greek yogurt
- 3 tablespoons chopped fresh mint
- 3 tablespoons extra-virgin olive oil
- 6 ounces cherry tomatoes, halved
- Salt and pepper

DIRECTIONS:
- Bring 4 quarts water to boil in a Dutch oven. Put in farro and 1 tablespoon salt, return to boil, and cook until grains are soft with slight chew, 15 to 30 minutes.
- Drain farro, spread in rimmed baking sheet, and allow to cool completely, about fifteen minutes.
- Beat oil, lemon juice, shallot, yogurt, ¼ teaspoon salt, and ¼ teaspoon pepper together in a big container.
- Put in farro, cucumber, tomatoes, arugula, and mint and toss gently to combine. Sprinkle with

salt and pepper to taste. Serve.
NUTRITION: Calories: 97 Carbs: 15g Fat: 4g Protein: 2g

Chorizo-Kidney Beans Quinoa Pilaf

Preparation time : 15 minutes
Cooking time : 37 minutes

Servings: 4

INGREDIENTS:

¼ pound dried Spanish chorizo diced (about 2/3 cup)
¼ teaspoon red pepper flakes
¼ teaspoon smoked paprika
½ teaspoon cumin
½ teaspoon sea salt
1 3/4 cups water
1 cup quinoa
1 large clove garlic minced
1 small red bell pepper finely diced
1 small red onion finely diced
1 tablespoon tomato paste
1 15-ounce can kidney beans rinsed and drained

DIRECTIONS:

Place a nonstick pot on medium high fire and heat for 2 minutes. Add chorizo and sauté for 5 minutes until lightly browned. Stir in peppers and onion. Sauté for 5 minutes.

Add tomato paste, red pepper flakes, salt, paprika, cumin, and garlic. Sauté for 2 minutes. Stir in quinoa and mix well. Sauté for 2 minutes.

Add water and beans. Mix well. Cover and simmer for 20 minutes or until liquid is fully absorbed.

Turn off fire and fluff quinoa. Let it sit for 5 minutes more while uncovered. Serve and enjoy.

NUTRITION: Calories: 260 Protein: 9.6g Carbs: 40.9g Fat: 6.8g

Goat Cheese 'N Red Beans Salad

Preparation time: 15 minutes

Cooking time: 0 minutes

Servings: 6

INGREDIENTS:

2 cans of Red Kidney Beans, drained and rinsed well

Water or vegetable broth to cover beans

1 bunch parsley, chopped

1 1/2 cups red grape tomatoes, halved

3 cloves garlic, minced

3 tablespoons olive oil

3 tablespoons lemon juice

1/2 teaspoon salt

1/2 teaspoon white pepper

6 ounces goat cheese, crumbled

DIRECTIONS:

In a large bowl, combine beans, parsley, tomatoes and garlic. Add olive oil, lemon juice, salt and pepper.

Mix well and refrigerate until ready to serve. Spoon into individual dishes topped with crumbled goat cheese.

NUTRITION: Calories: 385 Protein: 22.5g Carbs: 44.0g Fat: 15.0g

Greek Farro Salad

Preparation time : 15 minutes

Cooking time: 20 minutes

Servings: 4

INGREDIENTS:

Farro:

½ teaspoon fine-grain sea salt

1 cup farro, rinsed

1 tablespoon olive oil

2 garlic cloves, pressed or minced

Salad:

½ small red onion, chopped and then rinsed under water to mellow the flavor

1 avocado, sliced into strips

1 cucumber, sliced into thin rounds

15 pitted Kalamata olives, sliced into rounds

1-pint cherry tomatoes, sliced into rounds

2 cups cooked chickpeas (or one 14-ounce can, rinsed and drained)

5 ounces mixed greens

Lemon wedges

Herbed Yogurt Ingredients:

1/8 teaspoon salt

1 ¼ cups plain Greek yogurt

1 ½ tablespoon lightly packed fresh dill, roughly chopped

1 ½ tablespoon lightly packed fresh mint, torn into pieces

1 tablespoon lemon juice (about ½ lemon)

1 tablespoon olive oil

DIRECTIONS:

> In a blender, blend and puree all herbed yogurt ingredients and set aside. Then cook the farro by placing in a pot filled halfway with water.

> Bring to a boil, reduce fire to a simmer and cook for 15 minutes or until farro is tender. Drain well. Mix in salt, garlic, and olive oil and fluff to coat.

> Evenly divide the cooled farro into 4 bowls. Evenly divide the salad ingredients on the 4 farro bowl. Top with ¼ of the yogurt dressing. Serve and enjoy.

NUTRITION: Calories: 428 Protein: 17.7g Carbs: 47.6g Fat: 24.5g

White Bean and Tuna Salad

Preparation time: 15 minutes

Cooking time: 8 minutes

Servings : 4

INGREDIENT s:

- 1 (12 ounce) can solid white albacore tuna, drained
- 1 (16 ounce) can Great Northern beans, drained and rinsed
- 1 (2.25 ounce) can sliced black olives, drained
- 1 teaspoon dried oregano
- 1/2 teaspoon finely grated lemon zest
- 1/4 medium red onion, thinly sliced
- 3 tablespoons lemon juice
- 3/4-pound green beans, trimmed and snapped in half
- 4 large hard-cooked eggs, peeled and quartered
- 6 tablespoons extra-virgin olive oil
- Salt and ground black pepper, to taste

DIRECTIONS:

Place a saucepan on medium high fire. Add a cup of water and the green beans. Cover and cook for 8 minutes. Drain immediately once tender.

In a salad bowl, whisk well oregano, olive oil, lemon juice, and lemon zest. Season generously with pepper and salt and mix until salt is dissolved.

Stir in drained green beans, tuna, beans, olives, and red onion. Mix thoroughly to coat. Adjust seasoning to taste. Spread eggs on top. Serve and enjoy.

NUTRITION: Calories: 551 Protein: 36.3g Carbs: 33.4g Fat: 30.3g

Spicy Sweet Red Hummus

Preparation time : 15 minutes

Cooking time: 0 minutes

Servings: 8

INGREDIENTS:
- 1 (15 ounce) can garbanzo beans, drained
- 1 (4 ounce) jar roasted red peppers
- 1 1/2 tablespoons tahini
- 1 clove garlic, minced
- 1 tablespoon chopped fresh parsley
- 1/2 teaspoon cayenne pepper
- 1/2 teaspoon ground cumin
- 1/4 teaspoon salt
- 3 tablespoons lemon juice

DIRECTIONS:

In a blender, add all ingredients and process until smooth and creamy. Adjust seasoning to taste if needed. Can be stored in an airtight container for up to 5 days.

NUTRITION: Calories: 64 Protein: 2.5g Carbs: 9.6g Fat: 2.2g

Black Bean Chili with Mangoes

Preparation time: 15 minutes

Cooking time: 10 minutes

Servings: 4

INGREDIENTS:

    2 tablespoons coconut oil

    1 onion, chopped

    2 (15-ounce / 425-g) cans black beans, drained and rinsed

    1 tablespoon chili powder

    1 teaspoon sea salt

    ¼ teaspoon freshly ground black pepper

    1 cup water

    2 ripe mangoes, sliced thinly

    ¼ cup chopped fresh cilantro, divided

    ¼ cup sliced scallions, divided

DIRECTIONS:

Heat the coconut oil in a pot over high heat until melted. Put the onion in the pot and sauté for 5 minutes or until translucent.

Add the black beans to the pot. Sprinkle with chili powder, salt, and ground black pepper. Pour in the water. Stir to mix well.

Bring to a boil. Reduce the heat to low, then simmering for 5 minutes or until the beans are tender. Turn off the heat and mix in the mangoes, then garnish with scallions and cilantro before serving.

NUTRITION: Calories: 430 Fat: 9.1g Protein: 20.2g
Carbs: 71.9g

Israeli Style Eggplant and Chickpea Salad

Preparation time: 5 minutes

Cooking time: 20 minutes

Servings : 6

INGREDIENTS:

- 2 tablespoons balsamic vinegar
- 2 tablespoons freshly squeezed lemon juice
- 1 teaspoon ground cumin
- ¼ teaspoon sea salt
- 2 tablespoons olive oil, divided
- 1 (1-pound / 454-g) medium globe eggplant, stem removed, cut into flat cubes (about ½ inch thick)
- 1 (15-ounce / 425-g) can chickpeas, drained and rinsed
- ¼ cup chopped mint leaves
- 1 cup sliced sweet onion
- 1 garlic clove, finely minced
- 1 tablespoon sesame seeds, toasted

DIRECTIONS:

Preheat the oven to 550ºF (288ºC) or the highest level of your oven or broiler. Grease a baking sheet with 1 tablespoon of olive oil.

Combine the balsamic vinegar, lemon juice, cumin, salt, and 1 tablespoon of olive oil in a small bowl. Stir to mix well.

Arrange the eggplant cubes on the baking sheet, then brush with 2 tablespoons of the balsamic vinegar mixture on both sides.

Broil in the preheated oven for 8 minutes or until lightly browned. Flip the cubes halfway through the cooking time.

Meanwhile, combine the chickpeas, mint, onion, garlic, and sesame seeds in a large serving bowl. Drizzle with remaining balsamic vinegar mixture. Stir to mix well.

Remove the eggplant from the oven. Allow to cool for 5 minutes, then slice them into ½-inch strips on a clean work surface.

Add the eggplant strips in the serving bowl, then toss to combine well before serving.

NUTRITION: Calories: 125 Fat: 2.9g Protein: 5.2g Carbs: 20.9g

Italian Sautéed Cannellini Beans

Preparation time: 15 minutes

Cooking time: 15 minutes

Servings : 6

INGREDIENTS:

  2 teaspoons extra-virgin olive oil
  ½ cup minced onion
  ¼ cup red wine vinegar
  1 (12-ounce / 340-g) can no-salt-added tomato paste
  2 tablespoons raw honey
  ½ cup water
  ¼ teaspoon ground cinnamon
  2 (15-ounce / 425-g) cans cannellini beans

DIRECTIONS:

  Heat the olive oil in a saucepan over medium heat until shimmering. Add the onion and sauté for 5 minutes or until translucent.

  Pour in the red wine vinegar, tomato paste, honey, and water. Sprinkle with cinnamon. Stir to mix well.

  Reduce the heat to low, then pour all the beans into the saucepan. Cook for 10 more minutes. Stir constantly. Serve immediately.

NUTRITION: Calories: 435 Fat: 2.1g Protein: 26.2g Carbs: 80.3g

Lentil and Vegetable Curry Stew

Preparation time: 15 minutes
Cooking time: 4 hours & 7 minutes

Servings: 8

INGREDIENTS:

> 1 tablespoon coconut oil
> 1 yellow onion, diced
> ¼ cup yellow Thai curry paste
> 2 cups unsweetened coconut milk
> 2 cups dry red lentils, rinsed well and drained
> 3 cups bite-sized cauliflower florets
> 2 golden potatoes, cut into chunks
> 2 carrots, peeled and diced
> 8 cups low-sodium vegetable soup, divided
> 1 bunch kale, stems removed and roughly chopped
> Sea salt, to taste
> ½ cup fresh cilantro, chopped
> Pinch crushed red pepper flakes

DIRECTIONS:

> Heat the coconut oil in a nonstick skillet over medium-high heat until melted. Add the onion and sauté for 5 minutes or until translucent.
>
> Pour in the curry paste and sauté for another 2 minutes, then fold in the coconut milk and stir to combine well. Bring to a simmer and turn off the heat.
>
> Put the lentils, cauliflower, potatoes, and carrot in the slow cooker. Pour in 6 cups of vegetable

soup and the curry mixture. Stir to combine well.

Cover and cook on high for 4 hours or until the lentils and vegetables are soft. Stir periodically.

During the last 30 minutes, fold the kale in the slow cooker and pour in the remaining vegetable soup. Sprinkle with salt.

Pour the stew in a large serving bowl and spread the cilantro and red pepper flakes on top before serving hot.

NUTRITION: Calories: 530 Fat: 19.2g Protein: 20.3g Carbs: 75.2g

Lush Moroccan Chickpea, Vegetable, and Fruit Stew

Preparation time : 15 minutes
Cooking time: 6 hours & 4 minutes

Servings: 6

INGREDIENTS:

- 1 large bell pepper, any color, chopped
- 6 ounces (170 g) green beans, trimmed and cut into bite-size pieces
- 3 cups canned chickpeas, rinsed and drained
- 1 (15-ounce / 425-g) can diced tomatoes, with the juice
- 1 large carrot, cut into ¼-inch rounds
- 2 large potatoes, peeled and cubed
- 1 large yellow onion, chopped
- 1 teaspoon grated fresh ginger
- 2 garlic cloves, minced
- 1¾ cups low-sodium vegetable soup
- 1 teaspoon ground cumin
- 1 tablespoon ground coriander
- ¼ teaspoon ground red pepper flakes
- Sea salt and ground black pepper, to taste
- 8 ounces (227 g) fresh baby spinach
- ¼ cup diced dried figs
- ¼ cup diced dried apricots
- 1 cup plain Greek yogurt

DIRECTIONS:

Place the bell peppers, green beans, chicken peas, tomatoes and juice, carrot, potatoes, onion, ginger, and garlic in the slow cooker.

Pour in the vegetable soup and sprinkle with cumin, coriander, red pepper flakes, salt, and ground black pepper. Stir to mix well.

Put the slow cooker lid on and cook on high for 6 hours or until the vegetables are soft. Stir periodically. Open the lid and fold in the spinach, figs, apricots, and yogurt. Stir to mix well.

Cook for 4 minutes or until the spinach is wilted. Pour them in a large serving bowl. Allow to cool for at least 20 minutes, then serve warm.

NUTRITION: Calories: 611 Fat: 9.0g Protein: 30.7g Carbs: 107.4g

Lebanese Rice and Broken Noodles with Cabbage

Preparation time: 5 minutes

Cooking time: 25 minutes

Servings: 6

INGREDIENTS:

- 1 tablespoon extra-virgin olive oil
- 1 cup (about 3 ounces) uncooked vermicelli or thin spaghetti, broken into 1- to 1½-inch pieces
- 3 cups shredded cabbage (about half a 14-ounce package of coleslaw mix or half a small head of cabbage)
- 3 cups low-sodium or no-salt-added vegetable broth
- ½ cup water
- 1 cup instant brown rice
- 2 garlic cloves
- ¼ teaspoon kosher or sea salt
- 1/8 to ¼ teaspoon crushed red pepper
- ½ cup loosely packed, coarsely chopped cilantro
- Fresh lemon slices, for serving (optional)

DIRECTIONS:

In a large saucepan over medium-high heat, heat the oil. Add the pasta and cook for 3 minutes to toast, stirring often.

Add the cabbage and cook for 4 minutes, stirring often. Add the broth, water, rice, garlic, salt, and crushed red pepper, and bring to a boil over high heat.

Stir, cover, and reduce the heat to medium-low. Simmer for 10 minutes. Remove the pan from the heat, but do not lift the lid. Let sit for 5 minutes.

Fish out the garlic cloves, mash them with a fork, then stir the garlic back into the rice. Stir in the cilantro. Serve with the lemon slices (if using).

NUTRITION: Calories: 259 Fat: 4g Carbohydrates: 49g Protein: 7g

Lemon Farro Bowl with Avocado

Preparation time: 5 minutes

Cooking time: 25 minutes

Servings: 6

INGREDIENTS:

- 1 tablespoon plus 2 teaspoons extra-virgin olive oil, divided
- 1 cup chopped onion (about ½ medium onion)
- 2 garlic cloves, minced (about 1 teaspoon)
- 1 carrot, shredded (about 1 cup)
- 2 cups low-sodium or no-salt-added vegetable broth
- 1 cup (6 ounces) uncooked pearled or 10-minute farro
- 2 avocados, peeled, pitted, and sliced
- 1 small lemon
- ¼ teaspoon kosher or sea salt

DIRECTIONS:

In a medium saucepan over medium-high heat, heat 1 tablespoon of oil. Add the onion and cook for 5 minutes, stirring occasionally.

Add the garlic and carrot and cook for 1 minute, stirring frequently. Add the broth and farro, and bring to a boil over high heat.

Lower the heat to medium-low, cover, and simmer for about 20 minutes or until the farro is plump and slightly chewy (al dente).

Pour the farro into a serving bowl, and add the avocado slices. Using a Microplane or citrus zester, zest the peel of the lemon directly into the bowl of farro.

Halve the lemon, and squeeze the juice out of both halves using a citrus juicer or your hands. Drizzle the remaining 2 teaspoons of oil over the bowl, and sprinkle with salt. Gently mix all the ingredients and serve.

NUTRITION: Calories: 279 Fat: 14g Carbohydrates: 36g Protein: 7g

Barley Risotto with Parmesan

Preparation time: 5 minutes
Cooking time : 25 minutes

Servings: 6

INGREDIENTS:
- 4 cups low-sodium or no-salt-added vegetable broth
- 1 tablespoon extra-virgin olive oil
- 1 cup chopped yellow onion (about ½ medium onion)
- 2 cups uncooked pearl barley
- ½ cup dry white wine
- 1 cup freshly grated Parmesan cheese (about 4 ounces), divided
- ¼ teaspoon kosher or sea salt
- ¼ teaspoon freshly ground black pepper
- Fresh chopped chives and lemon wedges, for serving (optional)

DIRECTIONS:
Pour the broth into a medium saucepan and bring to a simmer. In a large stockpot over medium-high heat, heat the oil.

Add the onion and cook for 8 minutes, stirring occasionally. Add the barley and cook for 2 minutes, stirring until the barley is toasted.

Pour in the wine and cook for about 1 minute, or until most of the liquid evaporates. Add 1 cup of warm broth to the pot and cook, stirring, for about 2 minutes, or until most of the liquid is absorbed.

Add the remaining broth 1 cup at a time, cooking until each cup is absorbed (about 2 minutes each time) before adding the next. The last addition of broth will take a bit longer to absorb, about 4 minutes.

Remove the pot from the heat, and stir in ½ cup of cheese, and the salt and pepper. Serve with the remaining cheese on the side, along with the chives and lemon wedges (if using).

NUTRITION: Calories: 346 Fat: 7g Carbohydrates: 56g Protein: 14g

Garlic-Asparagus Israeli Couscous

Preparation time : 5 minutes

Cooking time: 25 minutes

Servings: 6

INGREDIENTS:

- 1 cup garlic-and-herb goat cheese (about 4 ounces)
- 1½ pounds asparagus spears, ends trimmed and stalks chopped into 1-inch pieces (about 2¾ to 3 cups chopped)
- 1 tablespoon extra-virgin olive oil
- 1 garlic clove, minced (about ½ teaspoon)
- ¼ teaspoon freshly ground black pepper
- 1¾ cups water
- 1 (8-ounce) box uncooked whole-wheat or regular

  Israeli couscous (about 1⅓ cups)

- ¼ teaspoon kosher or sea salt

DIRECTIONS:

Preheat the oven to 425°F. Put the goat cheese on the counter to bring to room temperature.

In a large bowl, mix together the asparagus, oil, garlic, and pepper. Spread the asparagus on a large, rimmed baking sheet and roast for 10 minutes, stirring a few times.

Remove the pan from the oven, and spoon the asparagus into a large serving bowl. While the asparagus is roasting, in a medium saucepan, bring the water to a boil.

Add the couscous and salt. Reduce the heat to medium-low, cover, and cook for 12 minutes, or until the water is absorbed.

Pour the hot couscous into the bowl with the asparagus. Add the goat cheese, mix thoroughly until completely melted, and serve.

NUTRITION: Calories: 263 Fat: 9g Carbohydrates: 36g Protein: 11g

Lentils with Spinach and Toasted Garlic

Preparation time: 10 minutes

Cooking time: 58 minutes

Servings: 6

INGREDIENTS:

- 2 tablespoons extra-virgin olive oil
- 4 garlic cloves, sliced thin
- Salt and pepper, to taste
- 1 onion, chopped fine
- 1 teaspoon ground coriander
- 1 teaspoon ground cumin
- 2½ cups water
- 1 cup green or brown lentils, picked over and rinsed
- 8 ounces (227 g) curly-leaf spinach, stemmed and chopped coarse
- 1 tablespoon red wine vinegar

DIRECTIONS:

Cook oil and garlic in large saucepan over medium-low heat, stirring often, until garlic turns crisp and golden but not brown, about 5 minutes.

Using slotted spoon, transfer garlic to paper towel–lined plate and season lightly with salt; set aside.

Add onion and ½ teaspoon salt to oil left in saucepan and cook over medium heat until softened and lightly browned, 5 to 7 minutes. Stir in coriander and cumin and cook until fragrant, about 30 seconds.

Stir in water and lentils and bring to simmer. Reduce heat to low, cover, and simmer gently, stirring occasionally, until lentils are mostly tender but still intact, 45 to 55 minutes.

Stir in spinach, 1 handful at a time. Cook, uncovered, stirring occasionally, until spinach is wilted and lentils are completely tender, about 8 minutes.

Stir in vinegar and season with salt and pepper to taste. Transfer to serving dish, sprinkle with toasted garlic, and serve.

NUTRITION: Calories: 160 Carbs: 22g Fat: 5g Protein: 8g

Stewed Oregano Chickpeas with Veggies

Preparation time: 15 minutes

Cooking time: 51 minutes

Servings: 6

INGREDIENTS:
- ¼ cup extra-virgin olive oil
- 2 onions, chopped
- 1 green bell pepper, stemmed, seeded, and chopped fine
- Salt and pepper, to taste
- 3 garlic cloves, minced
- 1 tablespoon minced fresh oregano or 1 teaspoon dried
- 2 bay leaves
- 1 pound (454 g) eggplant, cut into 1-inch pieces
- 1 (28-ounce / 794-g) can whole peeled tomatoes, drained with juice reserved, chopped coarse
- 2 (15-ounce / 425-g) cans chickpeas, drained with 1 cup liquid reserved

DIRECTIONS:
- Adjust oven rack to lower-middle position and heat oven to 400ºF (205ºC). Heat oil in Dutch oven over medium heat until shimmering.
- Add onions, bell pepper, ½ teaspoon salt, and ¼ teaspoon pepper and cook until softened, about 5 minutes. Stir in garlic, 1 teaspoon oregano, and bay leaves and cook until fragrant, about 30 seconds.

Stir in eggplant, tomatoes and reserved juice, and chickpeas and reserved liquid and bring to boil.

Transfer pot to oven and cook, uncovered, until eggplant is very tender, 45 to 60 minutes, stirring twice during cooking.

Discard bay leaves. Stir in remaining 2 teaspoons oregano and season with salt and pepper to taste. Serve.

NUTRITION: Calories: 133 Carbs: 20g Fat: 2g Protein: 7g

Hot Chickpeas with Turnips

Preparation time: 15 minutes

Cooking time: 31 minutes

Servings: 4-6

INGREDIENTS:

- 2 tablespoons extra-virgin olive oil
- 2 onions, chopped
- 2 red bell peppers, stemmed, seeded, and chopped
- Salt and pepper, to taste
- ¼ cup tomato paste
- 1 jalapeño chili, stemmed, seeded, and minced
- 5 garlic cloves, minced
- ¾ teaspoon ground cumin
- ¼ teaspoon cayenne pepper
- 2 (15-ounce / 425-g) cans chickpeas
- 12 ounces (340 g) turnips, peeled and cut into ½-inch pieces
- ¾ cup water, plus extra as needed
- ¼ cup chopped fresh parsley
- 2 tablespoons lemon juice, plus extra for seasoning

DIRECTIONS:

Heat oil in Dutch oven over medium heat until shimmering. Add onions, bell peppers, ½ teaspoon salt, and ¼ teaspoon pepper and cook until softened and lightly browned, 5 to 7 minutes.

Stir in tomato paste, jalapeño, garlic, cumin, and cayenne and cook until fragrant, about 30 seconds.

Stir in chickpeas and their liquid, turnips, and water. Bring to simmer and cook until turnips are tender and sauce has thickened, 25 to 35 minutes.

Stir in parsley and lemon juice. Season with salt, pepper, and extra lemon juice to taste. Adjust consistency with extra hot water as needed. Serve.

NUTRITION: Calories: 62 Carbs: 11g Fat: 2g Protein: 2g

Rich Chickpea Salad

Preparation time: 15 minutes
Cooking time : 3 minutes

Servings: 6

INGREDIENTS:

2 (15-ounce / 425-g) cans chickpeas, rinsed
¼ cup extra-virgin olive oil
2 tablespoons lemon juice
Salt and pepper, to taste
Pinch cayenne pepper
3 carrots, peeled and shredded
1 cup baby arugula, chopped coarse
½ cup pitted kalamata olives, chopped coarse

DIRECTIONS:

Microwave chickpeas in medium bowl until hot, about 2 minutes. Stir in oil, lemon juice, ¾ teaspoon salt, ½ teaspoon pepper, and cayenne and let sit for 30 minutes.

Add carrots, arugula, and olives and toss to combine. Season with salt and pepper to taste. Serve.

NUTRITION: Calories: 220 Carbs: 35g Fat: 6g Protein: 9g

Golden Falafel

Preparation time: 15 minutes

Cooking time: 6 minutes

Servings: 24

INGREDIENTS:
> Salt and pepper, to taste
> 12 ounces (340 g) dried chickpeas, picked over and rinsed
> 10 scallions, chopped coarse
> 1 cup fresh parsley leaves
> 1 cup fresh cilantro leaves
> 6 garlic cloves, minced
> ½ teaspoon ground cumin
> 1/8 teaspoon ground cinnamon
> 2 cups vegetable oil

DIRECTIONS:
> Dissolve 3 tablespoons salt in 4 quarts cold water in large container. Add chickpeas and soak at room temperature for at least 8 hours or up to 24 hours. Drain and rinse well.
>
> Process chickpeas, scallions, parsley, cilantro, garlic, 1 teaspoon salt, 1 teaspoon pepper, cumin, and cinnamon in food processor until smooth, about 1 minute, scraping down sides of bowl as needed.
>
> Pinch off and shape chickpea mixture into 2-tablespoon-size disks, about 1½ inches wide and 1 inch thick, and place on parchment paper–lined baking sheet. (Falafel can be refrigerated for up to 2 hours.)

Adjust oven rack to middle position and heat oven to 200°F (93°C). Set wire rack in rimmed baking sheet. Heat oil in 12-inch skillet over medium-high heat to 375°F (190°C).

Fry half of falafel until deep golden brown, 2 to 3 minutes per side. Adjust burner, if necessary, to maintain oil temperature of 375°F (190°C).

Using slotted spoon, transfer falafel to prepared sheet and keep warm in oven. Return oil to 375°F (190°C) and repeat with remaining falafel. Serve.

NUTRITION: Calories: 81 Carbs: 8g Fat: 3g Protein: 4g

Warm Spiced Cranberry Beans

Preparation time: 15 minutes
Cooking time : 1 hour & 30 minutes

Servings: 6-8

INGREDIENTS:

    Salt and pepper, to taste
    1 pound (454 g) dried cranberry beans, picked over and rinsed
    ¼ cup extra-virgin olive oil
    1 onion, chopped fine
    2 carrots, peeled and chopped fine
    4 garlic cloves, sliced thin
    1 tablespoon tomato paste
    ½ teaspoon ground cinnamon
    ½ cup dry white wine
    4 cups chicken or vegetable broth
    2 tablespoons lemon juice, plus extra for seasoning
    2 tablespoons minced fresh mint

DIRECTIONS:

Dissolve 3 tablespoons salt in 4 quarts cold water in large container. Add beans and soak at room temperature for at least 8 hours or up to 24 hours. Drain and rinse well.

Adjust oven rack to lower-middle position and heat oven to 350ºF (180ºC). Heat oil in Dutch oven over medium heat until shimmering.

Add onion and carrots and cook until softened, about 5 minutes. Stir in garlic, tomato paste, cinnamon, and ¼ teaspoon pepper and cook until fragrant, about 1 minute.

Stir in wine, scraping up any browned bits. Stir in broth, ½ cup water, and beans and bring to boil. Cover, transfer pot to oven, and cook until beans are tender, about 1½ hours, stirring every 30 minutes.

Stir in lemon juice and mint. Season with salt, pepper, and extra lemon juice to taste. Adjust consistency with extra hot water as needed. Serve.

NUTRITION: Calories: 205 Carbs: 24g Fat: 2g Protein: 16g

Ritzy Cranberry Beans

Preparation time: 15 minutes
Cooking time: 1 hour & 35 minutes

Servings: 6-8

INGREDIENTS:

Salt and pepper, to taste
1 pound (454 g) dried cranberry beans, picked over and rinsed
3 tablespoons extra-virgin olive oil
½ fennel bulb, 2 tablespoons fronds chopped, stalks discarded, bulb cored and chopped
1 cup plus 2 tablespoons red wine vinegar
½ cup sugar
1 teaspoon fennel seeds
6 ounces (170 g) seedless red grapes, halved
½ cup pine nuts, toasted

DIRECTIONS:

Dissolve 3 tablespoons salt in 4 quarts cold water in large container. Add beans and soak at room temperature for at least 8 hours or up to 24 hours. Drain and rinse well.

Bring beans, 4 quarts water, and 1 teaspoon salt to boil in Dutch oven. Reduce to simmer and cook, stirring occasionally, until beans are tender, 1 to 1½ hours. Drain beans and set aside.

Wipe Dutch oven clean with paper towels. Heat oil in now-empty pot over medium heat until shimmering.

Add fennel, ¼ teaspoon salt, and ¼ teaspoon pepper and cook until softened, about 5 minutes. Stir in 1 cup vinegar, sugar, and fennel seeds until sugar is dissolved.

Bring to simmer and cook until liquid is thickened to syrupy glaze and edges of fennel are beginning to brown, about 10 minutes.

Add beans to vinegar-fennel mixture and toss to coat. Transfer to large bowl and let cool to room temperature.

Add grapes, pine nuts, fennel fronds, and remaining 2 tablespoons vinegar and toss to combine. Season with salt and pepper to taste and serve.

NUTRITION: Calories: 147 Carbs: 44g Fat: 0g Protein: 15g

www.ingramcontent.com/pod-product-compliance
Lightning Source LLC
Chambersburg PA
CBHW050749030426
42336CB00012B/1728